Diabetes And Mental Health

Balancing Blood Sugar and Emotional Well-Being

By

Daniella Williams

Copyright © 2023 by Daniella Williams

All rights reserved. No part of this publication may be reproduced, distributed, or transmitted in any form or by any means, including photocopying, recording, or other electronic or mechanical methods, without the prior written permission of the publisher, except in the case of brief quotations embodied in critical reviews and certain other noncommercial uses permitted by copyright law.

TABLE OF CONTENT

Chapter 1: Introduction to Diabetes and Mental Health

In this initial chapter, we will go on a journey to investigate the delicate link between diabetes and mental health. Understanding this relationship is vital for anybody living with diabetes, whether as a patient, caregiver, or healthcare practitioner. This chapter tries to build the framework for the whole book by describing the key principles connected to diabetes and mental health.

1.1 Understanding Diabetes

Diabetes is a complicated and pervasive medical disorder that affects millions of persons globally. It is vital to know the foundations of diabetes before we go into its relationship with mental health.

1.1.1 What is Diabetes?

Diabetes, also referred to as diabetes mellitus, is a chronic metabolic illness characterized by increased amounts of glucose (sugar) in the blood. The body depends on a hormone called insulin to manage blood sugar. In diabetes, there is either inadequate insulin synthesis or defective use of insulin by the body's cells, resulting in high blood sugar levels.

1.1.2 Types of Diabetes

Diabetes is categorized into numerous kinds, including:

Type 1 Diabetes: An autoimmune condition where the body's immune system assaults and kills insulin-producing cells.

Type 2 Diabetes: Often connected to lifestyle factors, characterized by insulin resistance and inadequate insulin production.

Gestational Diabetes: Occurs throughout pregnancy and normally resolves after delivery.

Other Types: Less prevalent kinds of diabetes, such as monogenic and secondary diabetes.

1.1.3 Symptoms and Complications

The symptoms of diabetes might vary but usually include increased thirst, frequent urination, unexplained weight loss, and weariness. If left mismanaged, diabetes may lead to serious consequences, including heart disease, kidney damage, nerve difficulties, and eye impairment.

1.1.4 Diagnosis and Management

Diabetes is diagnosed by blood tests that detect glucose levels. Management often requires lifestyle adjustments (diet and exercise) and, in certain circumstances, drugs or insulin treatment.

1.2 The Link Between Diabetes and Mental Health

As we shift into the major issue of this book, it's crucial to realize the fundamental relationship between diabetes and mental health.

1.2.1 The Bidirectional Relationship

Diabetes and mental health are interwoven in a bidirectional interaction. On one side, diabetes may impair mental health by generating stress, worry, and sadness owing to the demands of treating the illness. On the other side, mental health conditions might impact blood sugar management and adherence to diabetic self-care.

1.2.2 Psychological Impact of Diabetes

Living with diabetes may be emotionally hard. The ongoing need for blood sugar testing, food restrictions, and medication management may contribute to stress and feelings of being overwhelmed. Over time, this might lead to mental health disorders such as sadness and anxiety.

1.2.3 Impact on Quality of Life

Mental health and diabetes are directly connected to an individual's total quality of life. When mental health is impaired, it may limit a person's capacity to properly manage their diabetes, leading to a cycle of declining physical and emotional well-being.

1.3 Purpose and Scope of the Book

This book seeks to give comprehensive insights, techniques, and support for persons confronting the twin difficulties of diabetes and mental health concerns.

1.3.1 Understanding the Complex Interplay

We will study the delicate relationship between diabetes and mental health, presenting a comprehensive knowledge of how one might impact the other.

1.3.2 Practical Guidance

Throughout this book, readers will get practical tips on managing diabetes and improving mental well-being. This covers ideas for stress management, keeping a healthy lifestyle, and seeking expert help.

1.3.3 Empowering Readers

Ultimately, our objective is to encourage readers to take charge of their health, both physically and psychologically. By the conclusion of this book, you will have a toolbox of knowledge and methods to lead a full life while controlling diabetes and maintaining your mental health.

As we continue our investigation of diabetes and mental health, realize that you are not alone in battling these issues. Together, we will navigate this path toward greater health and well-being.

Chapter 2: Types of Diabetes

Diabetes is a complicated disorder that affects millions of individuals globally. Understanding the various forms of diabetes is critical for efficient management and treatment. In this chapter, we'll cover the major kinds of diabetes, including Type 1 Diabetes, Type 2 Diabetes, Gestational Diabetes, and other less prevalent varieties.

2.1 Type 1 Diabetes

Type 1 Diabetes, sometimes referred to as juvenile diabetes, is an autoimmune disorder. In this kind, the immune system erroneously assaults and kills the insulin-producing cells in the pancreas. This leads to a significant insulin deficit, and the body cannot manage blood sugar levels adequately. Here's everything you need to know about Type 1 Diabetes:

Causes: The actual etiology of Type 1 Diabetes remains uncertain, however, it's likely to entail genetic and environmental factors.

Onset: It commonly develops in infancy or adolescence, however, it may occur at any age.

Symptoms: Common symptoms include increased thirst, frequent urination, unexplained weight loss, and intense exhaustion.

Treatment: People with Type 1 Diabetes need insulin injections or an insulin pump to maintain their blood sugar levels adequately.

Monitoring: Regular blood sugar monitoring is necessary to prevent problems. Continuous Glucose Monitoring (CGM) devices have grown more common.

Lifestyle: A balanced diet, frequent exercise, and stress management are vital for maintaining Type 1 Diabetes.

2.2 Type 2 Diabetes

Type 2 Diabetes is the most frequent kind of diabetes. It generally affects adults, however, it's growing increasingly widespread in younger groups due to lifestyle issues. Unlike Type 1 Diabetes, persons with Type 2 Diabetes still make insulin, but their systems do not utilize it properly. Here's a breakdown of Type 2 Diabetes:

Risk Factors: Obesity, poor nutrition, lack of physical exercise, and heredity are key risk factors for Type 2 Diabetes.

Signs: Early signs may be mild, such as repeated infections, poor wound healing, and increased thirst. Later symptoms might include weariness, impaired eyesight, and nerve damage.

Treatment: Management of Type 2 Diabetes frequently starts with lifestyle modifications, including weight reduction, a balanced diet, and regular exercise. Some patients may need oral medicines or insulin.

Consequences: If left untreated or inadequately managed, Type 2 Diabetes may lead to serious consequences, including heart disease, renal damage, and neuropathy.

2.3 Gestational Diabetes

Gestational Diabetes develops during pregnancy and is characterized by high blood sugar levels. It may impact the health of both the mother and the growing baby. Key points regarding Gestational Diabetes:

Risk Factors: Pregnancy-related hormonal changes may make some women more insulin-resistant. As a consequence, individuals may acquire Gestational Diabetes.

Screening: All pregnant women routinely have glucose tolerance testing to diagnose Gestational Diabetes.

Management: Most women may control Gestational Diabetes by dietary adjustments and frequent physical exercise. In rare circumstances, insulin may be necessary.

Risks: Untreated Gestational Diabetes may lead to difficulties during pregnancy and delivery, as well as an increased risk of Type 2 Diabetes for both the mother and child in the future.

2.4 Other Types of Diabetes

While Type 1, Type 2, and Gestational Diabetes are the most frequent kinds, there are additional, less prevalent types of diabetes. These include:

Monogenic Diabetes: Caused by a single gene mutation and commonly diagnosed in younger persons. Treatment differs depending on the exact genetic mutation.

Secondary Diabetes: Resulting from other health concerns, such as specific drugs, hormonal abnormalities, or pancreatic illnesses.

LADA (Latent Autoimmune Diabetes in Adults): A slow-progressing type of autoimmune diabetes that first presents as Type 2 Diabetes in adults.

MODY (Maturity-Onset Diabetes of the Young): A series of genetic abnormalities that produce diabetes in children and young people, commonly mistaken for Type 1 or Type 2 Diabetes.

Understanding these various types of diabetes is the first step in effectively managing the condition. Individuals with diabetes, their families, and healthcare professionals must tailor their approaches based on the specific type of diabetes in question. Proper management can significantly improve the quality of life for those living with diabetes.

Chapter 3: Understanding Mental Health

Mental health is a critical aspect of our overall well-being, and in this chapter, we will explore its definition, common mental health disorders, and the profound impact it has on our lives.

3.1 Defining Mental Health

3.1.1 What is Mental Health?

Mental health refers to our emotional, psychological, and social well-being. It encompasses our ability to handle stress, maintain healthy relationships, make sound decisions, and adapt to life's challenges. Good mental health is not merely the absence of mental illness but the presence of positive attributes like resilience, emotional stability, and a sense of purpose.

3.1.2 Factors Influencing Mental Health

Mental health is influenced by a combination of genetic, environmental, and lifestyle factors. Our early life events, such as trauma or abuse, may impact our mental health, as can our family history of mental health difficulties. Additionally, financial position, access to adequate healthcare, and general physical health are key factors in mental well-being.

3.1.3 Stigma Surrounding Mental Health

Unfortunately, mental health disorders have been stigmatized in many communities. This stigma might discourage persons from seeking assistance and support when required. It's crucial to overcome this stigma by promoting open and understanding talks about mental health.

3.2 Common Mental Health Disorders

3.2.1 Depression

Depression is one of the most frequent mental health conditions globally. It's characterized by persistent emotions of melancholy, despair, and a loss of interest in previously appreciated activities. Physical symptoms commonly accompany depression, such as changes in appetite, sleep difficulties, and exhaustion. Effective therapies, including counseling and medication, are available.

3.2.2 Anxiety Disorders

Anxiety disorders cover different ailments, including generalized anxiety disorder, panic disorder, and social anxiety disorder. These conditions feature extreme anxiety, dread, and anxiousness. Physical symptoms including heart palpitations, sweating, and shaking are typical. Anxiety disorders may greatly damage one's ability to lead a full life but can be treated with treatment and, in some situations, medication.

3.2.3 Bipolar Disorder

Bipolar disorder is characterized by significant mood fluctuations, from manic or hypomanic episodes (elevated mood, enhanced activity) to depressed periods (deep despair). These mood fluctuations may impair everyday living, relationships, and employment. Medication and treatment may help patients with bipolar illness retain stability.

3.2.4 Schizophrenia

Schizophrenia is a serious mental condition that affects a person's thoughts, emotions, and behavior. Symptoms may include hallucinations, delusions, and confused thinking. Treatment often includes antipsychotic drugs, counseling, and assistance from mental health specialists.

3.3 The Impact of Mental Health on Overall Well-being

3.3.1 Emotional Well-being

Good mental health is intimately connected to emotional well-being. It lets people experience a broad variety of emotions, understand and control them, and build resilience in the face of adversity. Individuals with great emotional well-being can deal with stress more efficiently.

3.3.2 Social Well-being

Mental health substantially impacts our social interactions. When we are psychologically well, we can create and sustain solid, supportive relationships. Conversely, untreated mental health illnesses may lead to social isolation and difficulty in connecting to others.

3.3.3 Cognitive Well-being

Cognitive well-being comprises our capacity to think rationally, make choices, and solve issues. Mental health issues may impede cognitive performance, making it hard to concentrate, recall, or make sensible decisions.

3.3.4 Physical Well-being

Physical and mental health are strongly interwoven. Mental health illnesses may affect physical health via stress-related symptoms, sleep disruptions, and changes in eating. Conversely, persistent physical ailments may influence mental health. Ensuring strong mental health is crucial for total physical well-being.

3.3.5 Occupational Well-being

Our mental health has a huge influence on our professional life. A healthy mind permits us to be productive, creative, and involved in our employment. On the contrary, mental health difficulties may lead to lower work performance, absenteeism, and even job termination.

In conclusion, knowing mental health is vital for living a full and balanced life. This chapter has defined mental health, addressed common mental health illnesses, and underlined its far-reaching influence on our entire well-being. By realizing the relevance of mental health and treating mental health concerns as they emerge, people may progress towards a better, happier life.

Chapter 4: Diabetes and Depression

Depression is a frequent and dangerous mental health problem that affects millions of individuals worldwide. When paired with diabetes, it may produce a complicated and stressful condition. In this chapter, we will study the confluence of diabetes and depression, with a specific emphasis on detecting the indications of depression in persons with diabetes, understanding the causes and risk factors, and finding effective therapy and management techniques.

4.1 Recognizing Depression in Individuals with Diabetes

Depression is not only a sensation of melancholy; it is a chronic and pervasive disorder that may profoundly influence a person's life. For patients with diabetes, detecting depression is of essential significance since it may impair their capacity to manage their illness efficiently.

Depression Symptoms: Common symptoms of depression include persistent feelings of melancholy, despair, and a loss of interest or pleasure in activities. Other indicators may include changes in eating and weight, sleep difficulties, exhaustion, trouble focusing, and even thoughts of self-harm or suicide.

Depression and Diabetes: The symptoms of depression might coincide with the everyday problems of controlling diabetes. This may lead to a hazardous loop where sadness makes it harder to control diabetes, and poorly managed diabetes can contribute to the development of depression.

Screening for Depression: Healthcare providers typically use questionnaires and interviews to test for depression in patients with diabetes. Being open and honest with your healthcare staff about your mental well-being is vital.

4.2 Causes and Risk Factors

Understanding the causes and risk factors for depression in adults with diabetes might give insight into why these two illnesses commonly coexist. Several things have a role:

Biological Factors: Diabetes may alter the brain and body in ways that may contribute to depression. Fluctuations in blood sugar levels may affect mood, and there may be a hereditary propensity for both diseases.

Psychological Factors: The stress of managing a chronic condition like diabetes, coping with complications, or fear of hypoglycemia may all contribute to the development of depression. Negative thinking habits and poor self-esteem might also play a role.

Social Factors: A lack of social support, isolation, and the stigma associated with diabetes may contribute to feelings of loneliness and melancholy. The stress of diabetes control may strain relationships and impact mental health.

Lifestyle Factors: Unhealthy lifestyle choices, such as a poor diet, lack of physical exercise, and drug misuse, may increase both diabetes and depression.

4.3 Treatment and Management Strategics

The good news is that depression in adults with diabetes is curable. It's necessary to approach therapy thoroughly and holistically:

Medication: Antidepressant drugs, such as selective serotonin reuptake inhibitors (SSRIs) or serotonin-norepinephrine reuptake inhibitors (SNRIs), are widely used to treat depressed symptoms.

Psychotherapy: Talk therapy, such as cognitive-behavioral therapy (CBT) or interpersonal therapy (IPT), may be particularly beneficial in helping patients with diabetes manage their depression. These treatments may address negative thinking patterns and provide coping methods.

Diabetes care: Proper diabetes care, including frequent monitoring of blood sugar levels, sticking to medication and insulin regimens, and a healthy lifestyle, may help ease symptoms of depression. Stable blood sugar levels may significantly improve mood.

Support Groups: Joining a support group for those with diabetes may create a sense of community and lessen feelings of loneliness. Sharing experiences and strategies with others may be empowering.

Self-Care: Self-care practices, including stress reduction techniques, regular exercise, a balanced diet, and adequate sleep, are crucial in controlling both diabetes and depression. These routines may promote physical and mental well-being.

Collaborative Care: Collaboration amongst healthcare providers, especially primary care doctors, endocrinologists, and mental health experts, is crucial in managing the twin issues of diabetes and depression.

In conclusion, depression and diabetes typically coexist, producing a complicated web of physical and mental issues. Recognizing the indications of depression, understanding its causes, and applying appropriate treatment and management techniques are critical stages in reclaiming control over your life and attaining greater mental and physical well-being. Remember, seeking treatment and support is a show of strength, and there is hope for a better future even while living with diabetes and depression.

Chapter 5: Diabetes and Anxiety

Anxiety is a frequent emotional reaction that many patients with diabetes feel. It's the sense of uneasiness, dread, or nervousness that may be expressed in numerous ways, from slight concern to severe panic. This chapter will dig into the complicated link between anxiety and diabetes, practical ways for dealing with diabetes-related anxiety, and the professional assistance available to help patients manage their anxiety successfully.

5.1 The Relationship Between Anxiety and Diabetes

Anxiety and diabetes frequently go hand in hand. Here, we'll investigate how these two requirements cross and impact one another.

5.1.1 Understanding the Connection

The relationship between anxiety and diabetes is complicated. People with diabetes may suffer anxiety for several causes, such as:

Daily Management Stresses: Managing diabetes involves regular attention to blood sugar readings, medication, and lifestyle variables including food and exercise. This constant duty may lead to chronic stress and, in turn, anxiety.

Fear of effects: The long-term effects of diabetes, such as heart disease, renal difficulties, and visual impairments, may be a cause of concern. Worries about these issues may lead to increased stress and anxiety.

Blood Sugar Swings: Fluctuations in blood sugar levels might create anxiety. Low blood sugar (hypoglycemia) may induce symptoms including shakiness and disorientation, which can be scary. On the other side, excessive blood sugar (hyperglycemia) may lead to weariness and irritation, which can also contribute to worry.

Social and Stigma-Related Concerns: People with diabetes may face social stigma or feel self-conscious about their disease. This might lead to worry and impair their mental health.

5.1.2 The Biological Mechanisms

Anxiety may also affect diabetes on a physiologic basis. Stress hormones, such as cortisol and adrenaline, are produced when we're nervous. These hormones may cause blood sugar levels to increase, which can be troublesome for persons with diabetes. Furthermore, worry might decrease insulin sensitivity, making it more tough to regulate blood sugar adequately.

5.2 Coping with Diabetes-Related Anxiety

Coping with anxiety is key to controlling diabetes efficiently. In this part, we'll cover practical techniques to assist folks in handling the emotional issues of diabetes.

5.2.1 Lifestyle Strategies

Regular Exercise: Physical exercise is a fantastic strategy to relieve anxiety. It helps produce endorphins, which are natural mood enhancers. Incorporating regular exercise into your routine may be an important technique in reducing anxiety.

Healthy Eating: Proper eating is vital for both diabetes control and mental wellness. A balanced diet that contains complex carbs, lean proteins, and healthy fats will help regulate blood sugar levels and decrease anxiety.

Stress-Reduction Techniques: Practices like meditation, deep breathing, and progressive muscle relaxation may help quiet the mind and decrease anxiety. Learning and integrating these skills into your everyday life may be incredibly useful.

5.2.2 Emotional Support

Social Support: Sharing your problems with friends and family might bring emotional comfort. Having a support system that understands your health and your anxieties may be a big source of relief.

Support Groups: Joining a diabetic support group may be tremendously beneficial. Interacting with people who have similar issues helps alleviate feelings of loneliness and worry.

Self-Monitoring: Keeping a record of your anxiety symptoms and triggers may help you detect trends and build coping methods.

5.3 Professional Support for Anxiety

Sometimes, diabetes-related anxiety may become overpowering, and professional help may be essential. In this part, we'll examine the different possibilities.

5.3.1 Mental Health Professionals

Therapists and Counselors: Mental health specialists, such as therapists and counselors, may help you handle the emotional elements of living with diabetes. They teach techniques to control anxiety and enhance your general mental well-being.

Psychiatrists: In certain circumstances, medication may be essential to treat anxiety properly. Psychiatrists may analyze your requirements and provide suitable drugs.

5.3.2 Diabetes Educators

Diabetes Educators: These experts specialize in educating patients with diabetes on how to manage their illness. They may give help in managing stress and anxiety associated with diabetes control.

5.3.3 Combining Care

In many circumstances, a combination of mental health assistance and diabetes education may be the most successful method. Working with a healthcare team that includes both mental health specialists and diabetes educators may offer complete treatment that addresses both the physical and emotional aspects of diabetes.

Managing anxiety while living with diabetes is a huge challenge, but it is manageable with the correct education and support. By recognizing the link between anxiety and diabetes, utilizing coping skills, and getting professional treatment when required, people may enhance their quality of life and successfully manage their diabetes.

Chapter 6: Diabetes and Stress

Stress is an inescapable part of life, and when you're living with diabetes, it may have a dramatic influence on your entire health. In this chapter, we'll cover stress, its impact on blood sugar, and, most importantly, ways to manage stress and develop resilience for improved diabetes control.

6.1 Understanding Stress and Its Effects on Blood Sugar

Stress is your body's natural reaction to a challenge or danger, whether actual or imagined. When you meet stress, your body produces chemicals, like cortisol and adrenaline, which prepare you to cope with the circumstance. In tiny, short-term doses, stress may be therapeutic. However, persistent stress may lead to several health concerns, particularly for persons with diabetes.

6.1.1 How Stress Affects Blood Sugar

When stress hormones spike in your body, they activate a "fight or flight" reaction. This reaction leads your liver to release stored glucose (sugar) into your circulation to give additional energy to your muscles and brain. This is your body's method of preparing for physical exercise, but it may also contribute to elevated blood sugar levels.

For persons with diabetes, this might be especially troublesome. If your body doesn't make enough insulin or doesn't utilize it efficiently (as is the situation in type 1 and type 2 diabetes), the increased glucose released into your circulation may cause a surge in blood sugar levels.

Chronic stress may also interrupt your food and exercise patterns, making it more tough to maintain your blood sugar levels. It could lead to bad coping techniques like emotional eating or missing meals, both of which can influence your diabetes control adversely.

6.1.2 Recognizing Stress Triggers

The first step in managing stress is knowing what provokes it. Common stresses might include work-related demands, financial difficulties, family challenges, health problems, and more. It's crucial to understand the origins of your stress so you can make proactive efforts to treat them.

6.2 Stress Management Techniques

Now that we've covered how stress impacts your blood sugar, let's go into effective stress management practices to help you keep better control of your diabetes.

6.2.1 Relaxation Techniques

Practicing relaxation methods may help decrease stress and minimize blood sugar increases. Techniques such as deep breathing techniques, gradual muscle relaxation, and meditation help quiet your mind and minimize the physiological stress reaction. You may integrate these routines into your everyday routine or employ them in stressful circumstances.

6.2.2 Physical Activity

Regular physical exercise is a potent stress buster. Exercise causes the production of endorphins, which are natural mood lifters. Additionally, it may assist in managing blood sugar levels. Aim for at least 150 minutes of moderate-intensity aerobic exercise each week, combined with muscle-strengthening activities on two or more days.

6.2.3 Healthy Eating Habits

Maintaining a well-balanced diet is vital for controlling stress. Avoid excessive intake of sugary or high-fat meals, since these may contribute to blood sugar spikes and falls. Focus on a diet rich in fruits, vegetables, whole grains, lean proteins, and healthy fats. Balanced eating may give consistent energy levels and improve stress management.

6.2.4 Time Management

Effective time management helps alleviate the stress associated with excessive schedules. Prioritize work, delegate where feasible, and establish reasonable targets. Break down major activities into smaller, doable stages to minimize feeling overwhelmed.

6.2.5 Seeking Social Support

Talking to friends, relatives, or a mental health professional may give emotional support during difficult times. Sharing your thoughts and worries with someone you trust may lessen stress and enhance your mental well-being.

6.3 Building Resilience for Better Diabetes Management

Building resilience is a critical component of managing diabetes and stress efficiently. Resilience is the capacity to adapt to and bounce back from hardship. Here are some ideas to help you become more resilient:

6.3.1 Education and Knowledge

Understanding your diabetes and how it interacts with stress is powerful. The more you know about your disease and its care, the better prepared you'll be to tackle stress-related issues.

6.3.2 Problem-Solving Skills

Develop problem-solving skills to manage the specific issues that diabetes-related stress might present. This can entail making a strategy for managing stress during holidays, job deadlines, or other high-stress circumstances.

6.3.3 Social Connections

Maintaining good social relationships might offer you a support network that can assist you in handling stress. Engage with support groups, friends, and family who understand your situation and can give emotional aid.

6.3.4 Positive Thinking

Fostering an optimistic mindset might boost your resilience. Practice positive self-talk and concentrate on your strengths. This approach may help you handle stress and diabetes with more confidence.

6.3.5 Adaptability

Remember that managing diabetes is a journey, and there will be ups and downs. Be flexible and adaptable in your approach, adjusting your diabetes management plan as needed.

In conclusion, managing stress is an integral part of effective diabetes care. By understanding how stress affects your blood sugar, implementing stress management techniques, and building resilience, you can take significant strides toward improving your overall health and well-being. It's important to remember that it's okay to seek help from healthcare professionals or mental health experts when needed, as they can provide valuable guidance and support in your journey to better manage diabetes-related stress.

Chapter 7: Diabetes Burnout

Dealing with diabetes daily can be incredibly challenging. From monitoring blood sugar levels to making dietary adjustments and taking medications, it's a constant juggling act. Amid this daily routine, many individuals with diabetes find themselves facing a phenomenon known as "diabetes burnout." This chapter explores what diabetes burnout is, how to recognize it, strategies for coping with it, and ways to prevent it to ensure you maintain good mental health while managing your diabetes.

7.1 Recognizing Diabetes Burnout

7.1.1 What is Diabetes Burnout?

Diabetes burnout is a state of emotional and mental exhaustion that often affects individuals living with diabetes. It's a feeling of being overwhelmed and fatigued by the constant demands of diabetes self-management. Diabetes burnout can manifest as frustration, hopelessness, and a lack of motivation to manage the condition effectively.

7.1.2 Signs of Diabetes Burnout

Recognizing diabetes burnout is essential to address it effectively. Here are some common signs and symptoms:

1. Neglecting Blood Sugar checking: People suffering from burnout could tend to overlook checking their blood sugar consistently, leading to poor management.

2. Unhealthy Eating Habits: An attitude of resignation may lead to poor nutritional

choices, further worsening blood sugar management.

3. Skipping prescriptions: Some persons may miss or forget to take their diabetic prescriptions, increasing the risk of complications.

4. Emotional Distress: Increased stress, worry, or depression may accompany diabetes burnout, making it much more tough to manage the illness.

5. Avoidance of Healthcare Providers: People may start skipping doctor's visits, which are crucial for effective diabetes control.

7.1.3 Understanding the Causes

Diabetes burnout may be induced by several circumstances, including:

stressful Self-Care Demands: The everyday chores of controlling diabetes, such as measuring blood sugar, taking medicines, and monitoring food intake, may become stressful.

Lack of Support: A lack of emotional and social support may lead to burnout.

Unrealistic Expectations: Setting unreasonably high expectations for oneself may lead to feelings of failure and weariness.

7.2 Strategies for Coping with Burnout

Coping with diabetes burnout is vital to recover control over your disease and enhance your general well-being. Here are some tips to help you handle diabetic burnout effectively:

1. Recognize and Accept: The first step is to recognize your burnout and accept it as a temporary difficulty. It's common to encounter these sensations at times.

2. Seek Support: Reach out to your healthcare team, friends, and family for emotional support. Talking to someone who knows your challenges may be incredibly beneficial.

3. Set Realistic objectives: Reevaluate your diabetes management objectives. Set manageable, realistic aims to decrease the strain you take on yourself.

4. Take occasional pauses: It's good to take occasional pauses from diabetes treatment. But ensure these breaks are planned and temporary to avoid long-term complications.

5. Self-Care: Prioritize self-care by engaging in activities that relax and rejuvenate you.

This can include exercise, meditation, hobbies, or spending time with loved ones.

6. Professional Help: If your burnout is severe, consider seeking professional help from a therapist or counselor who specializes in diabetes-related emotional issues.

7.3 Preventing Burnout in Diabetes Management

Preventing diabetes burnout is always better than dealing with it after it has taken hold. Here's how you can work on preventing burnout:

1. Education: Continuously educate yourself about diabetes management. The more you understand your condition, the better equipped you are to handle it.

2. Emotional Support: Build a strong support system of friends and family who

can provide emotional support when you need it.

3. Regular Check-Ins: Maintain regular check-ins with your healthcare practitioner. Discuss any emotional or mental health issues as part of your usual treatment.

4. Set limits: Learn to say no when you need to, and set limits to safeguard your mental and emotional well-being.

5. Seek a Diabetes Educator: Consider working with a qualified diabetes educator who can give direction and assistance for diabetes management.

In summary, diabetes burnout is a typical difficulty that persons with diabetes may encounter. Recognizing it is the first step towards conquering it, and numerous tactics may help you handle and avoid burnout. By taking care of your mental health and emotional well-being, you may have a full life while managing your diabetes efficiently. Remember, you're not alone in this path, and with the correct assistance and methods, you can reclaim control over your condition.

Chapter 8: Eating Disorders and Diabetes

8.1 The Intersection of Eating Disorders and Diabetes

Eating disorders and diabetes frequently cross, providing a hard dual diagnosis for people afflicted. In this chapter, we will investigate how these two illnesses connect and the particular complications they add to an individual's physical and emotional well-being.

Eating disorders, such as anorexia nervosa, bulimia nervosa, and binge-eating disorder, are characterized by poor eating behaviors and a distorted body image. These illnesses may co-occur with diabetes, both type 1 and type 2. The interaction of eating disorders with diabetes is complicated and possibly life-threatening since it affects blood sugar regulation and general health.

8.2 Identifying Signs of Eating Disorders

Recognizing the indicators of eating disorders in persons with diabetes is critical for early intervention and support. Here, we look into the general symptoms of eating disorders and the unique issues experienced by persons with diabetes.

Excessive Weight Loss: One of the first indicators is unexplained and severe weight loss. In those with diabetes, this may further disturb blood sugar management, leading to significant health consequences.

Preoccupation with Food: People with eating disorders typically obsess over food, monitoring calories, and indulging in ritualistic eating patterns. This fixation might affect diabetes control, producing blood sugar swings.

Purging Behaviors: Frequent use of laxatives, diuretics, or forced vomiting is frequent in various eating disorders. This may produce electrolyte imbalances, harming both physical and mental health.

Food Hoarding or Bingeing: Individuals may eat excessive quantities of food during binge episodes, followed by feelings of guilt or shame. Managing blood sugar in such instances becomes unpredictable.

Excessive Exercise: Over-exercising may be a hallmark of some eating disorders, and this intensive physical activity can disrupt diabetes control.

Isolation and Social Withdrawal: People with eating disorders may withdraw themselves owing to fear of criticism, making it vital to treat the emotional elements of these problems.

8.3 Treatment and Support for Dual Diagnosis

Dual diagnosis of eating disorders and diabetes demands a comprehensive strategy to treat both physical and mental health requirements. This section focuses on techniques for successful treatment and support.

Medical Intervention: Medical experts, including endocrinologists, nutritionists, and mental health specialists, cooperate to establish a specific treatment plan. They monitor blood sugar management while managing the eating issue.

Nutritional Counseling: A licensed dietitian plays a vital role in helping patients with diabetes and eating disorders build a balanced relationship with food. Balancing dietary demands and psychological well-being is crucial.

Therapeutic Approaches: Psychotherapy, such as cognitive-behavioral therapy (CBT) and dialectical-behavior therapy (DBT), may help persons with eating disorders address underlying emotional difficulties while developing coping mechanisms.

Support Groups: Group treatment sessions give a forum for people to discuss their experiences, struggles, and accomplishments with others suffering from similar dual conditions.

Family Involvement: In many circumstances, including the family is important for a successful rehabilitation. Family members may assist and obtain a deeper understanding of their loved one's problems.

Medication Management: In certain situations, psychiatric drugs may be administered to treat co-occurring mental health issues, such as depression or anxiety, that typically accompany eating disorders.

Continuous Monitoring: Long-term follow-up and monitoring are important to maintain sustained recovery and appropriate diabetes control. Regular check-ins with healthcare specialists help monitor improvement.

Education and Awareness: Raising awareness of the connection between eating disorders and diabetes is vital for early identification and decreasing stigma. Education may empower people to seek treatment and foster a supportive community.

Self-Management Methods: Equipping people with appropriate self-management methods for both diabetes and eating disorders is crucial to preserving their well-being over time.

In conclusion, the junction of eating disorders and diabetes is a difficult problem that demands comprehensive and multidisciplinary treatment. Early detection and intervention, together with continuous care, play essential roles in helping persons with multiple illnesses recover control of their lives and achieve greater physical and mental health. The route to recovery is tough, but with the correct therapy and support, it is possible to overcome these linked diseases and enjoy a full life.

Chapter 9: Diabetes and Cognitive Function

Cognitive function, which covers memory, reasoning, and decision-making skills, plays a critical part in our everyday lives. In this chapter, we study the complicated link between diabetes and cognitive health. We'll examine how diabetes may impair cognitive function, give measures for preserving brain health, and address the cognitive issues that persons with diabetes could confront.

9.1 Impact of Diabetes on Cognitive Health

Diabetes isn't restricted to influencing blood sugar levels; it may also have far-reaching implications on cognitive function. This section explores the different ways in which diabetes might impair our cognitive ability.

9.1.1 Cognitive Decline

One of the key concerns for patients with diabetes is the increased risk of cognitive impairment. Studies have indicated that poorly controlled diabetes, particularly in older persons, is related to an increased probability of acquiring illnesses such as Alzheimer's disease and vascular dementia.

9.1.2 Blood Sugar Fluctuations

The volatility in blood sugar levels, frequent in untreated diabetes, may contribute to cognitive problems. Frequent periods of high or low blood sugar may induce disorientation, trouble focusing, and memory lapses.

9.1.3 Blood Vessel Damage

Diabetes may damage blood arteries, particularly those in the brain. This vascular injury may limit blood supply to the brain, reducing cognitive function.

9.1.4 Inflammation

Chronic inflammation, frequently observed in diabetes, may significantly influence the brain. It may contribute to cognitive issues by activating an inflammatory reaction in the brain.

9.1.5 Insulin Resistance

Insulin, a hormone involved in blood sugar management, also plays a key role in brain function. Insulin resistance, frequent in type 2 diabetes, might interfere with insulin's effects in the brain, possibly leading to cognitive difficulties.

9.2 Strategies for Maintaining Brain Health

Fortunately, there are various treatments to assist in preserving and even enhancing cognitive function in adults with diabetes.

9.2.1 Blood Sugar Management

The cornerstone of cognitive health in diabetes is adequate blood sugar control. Regular monitoring, adherence to medication or insulin regimens, and a balanced diet may help stabilize blood sugar levels.

9.2.2 Healthy Eating

A diet rich in nutrients, particularly antioxidants and omega-3 fatty acids, may boost brain function. Foods like leafy greens, berries, and seafood may be healthy.

9.2.3 Physical Activity

Regular exercise is not only vital for treating diabetes but also for boosting brain health. Physical exercise boosts blood flow to the brain and may help lower the risk of cognitive deterioration.

9.2.4 Mental Stimulation

Challenging your brain with hobbies like puzzles, reading, or learning a new skill may assist in sustaining cognitive function. This mental activity may create and strengthen brain connections.

9.2.5 Stress Management

Stress may increase cognitive issues. Techniques such as meditation, mindfulness, and relaxation exercises may assist in managing stress and safeguard cognitive health.

9.3 Cognitive Challenges in Diabetes Management

Managing diabetes comes with its share of cognitive problems, and being aware of these barriers is vital for good self-care.

9.3.1 Medication Management

Taking drugs on schedule and in the exact dosages may be challenging, particularly for persons who may have memory challenges. Using medicine reminders or pill organizers may help.

9.3.2 Blood Sugar Monitoring

Frequent blood sugar monitoring takes attention and organization. Recording outcomes and spotting trends is critical for good diabetes treatment.

9.3.3 Decision-Making

Individuals with diabetes typically need to make rapid judgments regarding dietary choices, insulin dosages, and physical exercise. Cognitive function is key in making these judgments.

9.3.4 Coping with Diabetes-Related Stress

The everyday duties of controlling diabetes may be psychologically draining. Coping with stress and preventing burnout are cognitive issues that people must confront.

In conclusion, diabetes and cognitive function are tightly related. Managing diabetes well via blood sugar control, a healthy lifestyle, and stress management may considerably lessen the effects on cognitive health. Additionally, being cognizant of the cognitive hurdles inherent to diabetes care might enable people to better negotiate the intricacies of living with this illness while protecting their cognitive well-being.

Chapter 10: Social and Emotional Aspects of Diabetes

Diabetes is not merely a medical ailment; it has severe social and emotional repercussions. In this chapter, we will go into the subtleties of how diabetes impacts your relationships, how to manage stigma and prejudice, and the need to develop a supportive social network to aid you on your diabetes journey.

10.1 Navigating Relationships with Diabetes

Living with diabetes may have a big influence on your relationships. It's crucial to negotiate these connections with care and compassion. Here are some crucial aspects to consider:

10.1.1 Communication is Key

Effective communication is the basis of every healthy relationship. Discuss your diabetes with your loved ones, describing what it means for your everyday life and how they can help you. Open, honest interactions help eliminate misconceptions and develop empathy.

10.1.2 Involving Your Partner

If you have a partner, include them in your diabetes treatment. They may be a fantastic source of assistance, particularly when you need help monitoring your blood sugar, making balanced meals, or even simply emotional support during challenging times.

10.1.3 Friends and Family

Friends and family may also play a vital influence. Educate them about diabetes, so they may better grasp the obstacles you experience. Don't hesitate to depend on them when you need aid or encouragement.

10.2 Addressing Stigma and Discrimination

Diabetes, unfortunately, bears a stigma in society. Many individuals have misunderstandings about the disease, which may lead to prejudice. Addressing stigma and prejudice is vital for your emotional well-being:

10.2.1 Educating Others

One method to overcome stigma is via education. Correct misunderstandings about diabetes and share your experiences with others. The more people understand, the less likely they are to judge or discriminate against you.

10.2.2 Self-Empowerment

Believe in your power and ability. Refuse to allow the stigma around diabetes to impair your self-esteem. You are not defined by your situation, and you may have a full life.

10.2.3 Legal Rights

Know your legal rights against discrimination due to diabetes. Laws exist to safeguard those with chronic diseases. If you suffer prejudice, don't hesitate to take legal remedies.

10.3 Building a Supportive Social Network

A solid support system is crucial in treating diabetes and preserving your mental well-being:

10.3.1 Diabetes Support Groups

Join local or online diabetic support groups. These groups may provide a lot of knowledge, emotional support, and a feeling of belonging.

10.3.2 Mental Health Professionals

Consider consulting with a mental health professional, such as a therapist or counselor. They can assist you in negotiating the emotional elements of diabetes and give coping methods.

10.3.3 Building New Relationships

Don't be hesitant to meet new folks who have similar experiences. Building new connections within the diabetic community may be both soothing and inspiring.

10.3.4 Self-Care

Remember that self-care is not selfish. Take time for yourself, participate in things you like, and prioritize your mental health. A well-cared-for mind will assist your diabetes control.

10.3.5 Allies in Your Journey

Identify folks in your life who support you. Nurture these connections, as they may be your friends in the battle against diabetes-related stress and emotional issues.

In conclusion, navigating the social and emotional components of diabetes might be as crucial as controlling the medical parts of the illness. Effective communication, education, and support may help you maintain healthy relationships, overcome stigma and prejudice, and establish a powerful network to assist you in your diabetes journey. Remember, you're not alone, and with the appropriate attitude, diabetes can be controlled while protecting your mental well-being.

Chapter 11: Diabetes Self-Care and Mental Health

Living with diabetes may be a hard and challenging process. It entails not just the regulation of blood sugar levels but also a complex balance between physical health and emotional well-being. This chapter covers how to negotiate the complexity of self-care while keeping a pleasant and stable mental state.

11.1 Balancing Diabetes Self-Care and Mental Well-being

Living with diabetcs frequently entails balancing multiple duties, including checking blood sugar, taking medicines, and adopting smart lifestyle choices. However, these regular duties may occasionally take a toll on your mental health. In this part, we'll examine the delicate balance between diabetic self-care and mental well-being.

Understanding the Connection: To strike a balance, it's vital to realize the symbiotic link between physical and mental health. Fluctuations in blood sugar levels may alter mood, whereas stress and emotions can influence blood sugar. Understanding this link is the first step.

Accepting Imperfection: It's crucial to realize that diabetes treatment isn't about perfection. You will have good days and not-so-good days. Give yourself the freedom to make errors without feeling guilty. It's part of the process.

Stress Management: Stress is a typical companion of diabetes, and it may have a severe influence on your mental health. Learning appropriate stress management practices, such as deep breathing, meditation, or mindfulness, may help keep stress in control.

Seeking help: Don't hesitate to seek emotional help. Whether it's via friends, family, a therapist, or a support group, having someone to speak to helps reduce the emotional load of diabetes control.

11.2 Practical Tips for Self-Care

Effective self-care is the cornerstone of diabetic control. It not only helps you maintain better physical health but also adds to a healthy mood. Here are some practical strategies for self-care:

Healthy Eating: Focus on a balanced diet rich in vegetables, fruits, lean meats, and whole grains. Monitor your carbohydrate consumption, but also allow yourself occasional pleasures.

Regular Physical Activity: Exercise has a twofold advantage. It helps manage blood sugar levels and produces endorphins that boost your mood. Find an activity you like to make it a lasting habit.

Medication Adherence: Ensure you take your prescription medicines as instructed by your healthcare professional. Medication non-adherence may lead to variations in blood sugar levels, which might influence your emotional well-being.

Blood Sugar Monitoring: Regularly check your blood sugar levels, but don't allow the numbers to determine your value. Understand that some fluctuation is natural, and patterns are more essential than single data.

Adequate Sleep: Prioritize quality sleep. Poor sleep may alter blood sugar management and contribute to increased stress and irritability.

11.3 Goal Setting for a Healthy Mind and Body

Setting reasonable objectives might help you maintain both physical and emotional health. Here's how to do it:

SMART Objectives: Use the SMART (Specific, Measurable, Achievable, Relevant, Time-bound) criteria while defining objectives. For example, make a goal to walk for 30 minutes a day, five days a week.

Break It Down: Divide big tasks into smaller, doable stages. This makes the journey to your objective less daunting.

Track Progress: Keep a diary to document your progress. This not only helps you keep responsible but also enables you to see how far you've come.

Reward Yourself: Celebrate your victories, no matter how modest they may appear. Rewards may be a tremendous motivator.

Flexibility: Be flexible and change your objectives as required. Life is full of surprises, and it's normal to alter your objectives to changing circumstances.

Balancing diabetic self-care and mental well-being is a continuous endeavor. The goal is to retain an optimistic outlook, accept the rare setbacks, and keep going ahead. With the correct self-care practices and reasonable objectives, you may flourish while controlling diabetes and keeping a healthy mind and body. Remember, you're not alone on this road, and seeking help is a show of strength, not weakness.

Chapter 12: Diabetes and Sleep

12.1 The Bidirectional Relationship Between Diabetes and Sleep

Sleep is a key element of our lives, affecting both our physical and mental well-being. When it comes to diabetes, the association between sleep and the illness is bidirectional, meaning that diabetes may impact sleep, and sleep can affect diabetes. In this part, we will look into the subtle relationships between diabetes and sleep.

12.1.1 How Diabetes Affects Sleep

Blood Sugar Variations: One of the key ways diabetes affects sleep is via blood sugar variations. High blood sugar levels, a characteristic of diabetes, may lead to frequent urine throughout the night (nocturia). This may disturb sleep habits and contribute to sleep deprivation.

Neuropathy and Restless Legs: Diabetic neuropathy, which causes numbness and tingling in the limbs, may be aggravated at night, leading to pain and restless legs syndrome. These feelings might make it tough to fall and remain asleep.

Sleep Apnea: Type 2 diabetes is closely connected to sleep apnea, a disease when breathing is intermittently disrupted during sleep. Sleep apnea is typically caused by obesity, which is a significant risk factor for type 2 diabetes.

12.1.2 How Sleep Affects Diabetes

Insulin Sensitivity: Adequate sleep is vital for maintaining insulin sensitivity. Sleep loss may contribute to insulin resistance, making blood sugar management more problematic for those with diabetes.

Hormone Regulation: Sleep is vital for regulating hormones that impact hunger and metabolism. Poor sleep may contribute to overeating and weight increase, which are risk factors for type 2 diabetes.

Stress and Mental Health: Sleep deficiency may raise stress and damage mental health. Managing diabetes typically demands a great lot of emotional fortitude, and inadequate sleep may make it more difficult to cope with the everyday difficulties.

12.2 Strategies for Improving Sleep Quality

Now that we understand the deep link between diabetes and sleep, it's vital to study techniques for enhancing sleep quality, which may eventually aid in controlling diabetes more successfully.

12.2.1 Sleep Hygiene

Consistent Sleep Schedule: Try to go to bed and get up at the same times every day, especially on weekends. This helps adjust your body's internal clock.

Create a suitable Sleep Environment: Ensure your bedroom is dark, quiet, and at a suitable temperature. Invest in a comfy mattress and pillows.

Limit Exposure to Displays: The blue light from displays (phones, tablets, laptops, TVs) might interfere with your body's generation of melatonin, a hormone that controls sleep. Avoid screens at least one hour before sleep.

12.2.2 Lifestyle Modifications

Regular Exercise: Engaging in regular physical exercise may promote better sleep. Aim for at least 30 minutes of activity most days, but avoid severe exercise close tonight.

Balanced Diet: Maintaining a balanced diet may help manage blood sugar levels and promote sleep. Avoid large meals and coffee before night.

Tension Management: Practice relaxation methods such as deep breathing, meditation, or yoga to decrease tension and anxiety that might interfere with sleep.

12.3 Sleep Disorders in Diabetes

Diabetes may also make patients more prone to certain sleep disturbances. Understanding these illnesses is vital for addressing both ailments properly.

12.3.1 Sleep Apnea

Understanding Sleep Apnea: Sleep apnea is characterized by periodic pauses in breathing during sleep. It is more frequent in patients with type 2 diabetes.

Diagnosis and Treatment: If you suspect sleep apnea, it's vital to visit a healthcare expert for a diagnosis. Treatment treatments may include lifestyle adjustments, CPAP (Continuous Positive Airway Pressure) therapy, or surgery.

12.3.2 Insomnia

Insomnia and Diabetes: Insomnia entails difficulties getting asleep or staying asleep. Stress associated with diabetes care might lead to sleeplessness.

Addressing Insomnia: Cognitive-behavioral therapy for insomnia (CBT-I) is an evidence-based technique to treat insomnia. This treatment may help patients build healthy sleep habits and lessen anxiety connected to sleep.

12.3.3 Restless Legs Syndrome (RLS)

RLS in Diabetics: RLS is a disorder where patients suffer pain and an uncontrolled need to move their legs, often during the night. Diabetic neuropathy might worsen RLS symptoms.

Treatment Options: Treatment for RLS may entail lifestyle modifications, medicines, and regulating blood sugar levels to relieve neuropathy symptoms.

Understanding the complicated link between diabetes and sleep and applying methods for improved sleep hygiene and lifestyle adjustments is critical for those with diabetes. By enhancing sleep quality, you may favorably improve your blood sugar control and general well-being, making the treatment of diabetes more manageable and less burdensome on your mental health.

Chapter 13: Mindfulness and Diabetes

In the fast-paced world we live in, treating a chronic disease like diabetes may often seem overwhelming. The ongoing need to check blood sugar levels, take medicines, and make dietary modifications may be stressful. This is where mindfulness, a practice strongly founded in ancient traditions, may be a useful tool in your diabetes control toolkit. In this chapter, we'll examine the significant advantages of mindfulness in diabetes management, how to integrate mindfulness practices into your daily routine, and the fundamental notion of mindful eating for improved blood sugar control.

13.1 Benefits of Mindfulness in Diabetes Management

Mindfulness, in the context of diabetes treatment, is the discipline of remaining completely present and engaged at the moment without judgment. It entails being aware of your thoughts, emotions, physiological sensations, and the world around you. The advantages of mindfulness in diabetes control are many and may dramatically boost your well-being:

Stress Reduction: Stress is a typical companion for persons living with diabetes. Mindfulness practices, such as deep breathing and meditation, may help lower stress levels, which, in turn, can contribute to improved blood sugar management.

Improved Emotional Health: Mindfulness helps enhance emotional control and minimize feelings of anxiety and sadness typically linked with diabetes.

Enhanced Blood Sugar Management: By promoting awareness of your body, mindfulness may help you notice early indicators of high or low blood sugar, allowing for timely treatments.

Better Decision Making: Being present and attentive may help you make better choices in terms of nutrition, exercise, and general self-care.

Increased Adherence: Mindfulness may boost your adherence to your diabetes treatment practice. When you're present at the moment, you're more likely to follow your recommended meds and food programs.

Enhanced Quality of Life: Mindfulness may boost your overall quality of life by helping you concentrate on the good parts of life and creating a feeling of appreciation.

13.2   Incorporating   Mindfulness Practices

Incorporating mindfulness activities into your everyday routine doesn't have to be scary or time-consuming. Here are some basic methods to get started:

Meditation: Meditation is one of the most well-known mindfulness techniques. You may start with small workouts, perhaps as brief as 5-10 minutes a day. Find a peaceful, comfortable position, shut your eyes, and concentrate on your breath. When your mind wanders (as it certainly will), gently bring your focus back to your breath.

Deep Breathing: A brief deep breathing practice may be done anywhere. Take a few seconds to take in deeply with your nose, hold your breath momentarily, and then exhale slowly through your mouth. This simple activity might help relax your mind and lessen tension.

Body Scan: A body scan entails mentally "scanning" your body from head to toe, paying attention to any tension or pain. This exercise might help you become more aware of bodily feelings and identify areas of stress.

Mindful Walking: Walking may be a mindfulness activity. As you walk, pay attention to each step, the feeling of your feet striking the ground, and the sense of movement. This may be done inside or outdoors.

Yoga: Yoga blends physical postures with concentration and regulated breathing. There are numerous forms of yoga, so you may select one that matches your fitness level and interests.

13.3 Mindful Eating and Blood Sugar Control

When it comes to diabetes, what you eat and how you eat may have a big influence on your blood sugar levels. Mindful eating means being completely present throughout meals, making conscious decisions, and appreciating each mouthful. Here's how mindful eating may help you maintain improved blood sugar control:

Meal Control: Mindful eating may help you become more conscious of meal proportions. By paying attention to your body's hunger and fullness signals, you may prevent overeating and better regulate your blood sugar.

Slower Eating: Eating slowly enables your body to metabolize food more effectively, which may help reduce blood sugar increases.

Choosing Nutrient-Dense Foods: When you're attentive to your meal choices, you're more likely to pick healthy foods that promote stable blood sugar levels.

Blood Sugar Monitoring: Mindful eating entails monitoring how various meals influence your blood sugar. This knowledge may help you make smart eating decisions.

Stress Reduction: Eating mindfully may decrease stress, which, as discussed previously, is a major element in blood sugar regulation.

In summary, mindfulness is a significant tool in diabetes treatment. It provides several advantages, including stress reduction, greater mental well-being, and enhanced blood sugar management. By adding mindfulness techniques into your daily routine and practicing mindful eating, you may enhance your overall health and well-being while efficiently managing your diabetes.

Chapter 14: Exercise, Diabetes, and Mental Health

Physical activity and exercise have a significant role in the treatment of diabetes. In this chapter, we'll investigate the multidimensional link between exercise, diabetes, and mental health. We'll go into the science behind how exercise affects blood sugar regulation, and its function as a mood regulator, and give practical recommendations for building an exercise regimen that is both successful and pleasurable.

14.1 The Role of Exercise in Diabetes Management

Managing diabetes includes a precise balance between blood sugar management, medicine (if needed), and lifestyle factors.

Exercise is a strong tool in this equation for various reasons:

A. Improved Insulin Sensitivity: When you participate in physical exercise, your muscles require more glucose for energy. This causes your cells to become more receptive to insulin, making it simpler for your body to control blood sugar levels.

B. Blood Sugar Control: Regular exercise helps normalize blood sugar levels. It decreases insulin resistance, which is a prevalent problem in type 2 diabetes and may lead to more regular blood sugar readings.

C. Weight Management: Exercise helps with weight reduction or maintenance. Excess body weight is a key risk factor for type 2 diabetes, and reducing pounds may improve blood sugar management.

D. Cardiovascular Health: Diabetes raises the risk of heart disease. Exercise helps enhance cardiovascular health, lowering the risk of issues connected to the heart and blood vessels.

E. Stress Reduction: Stress may severely affect blood sugar levels. Exercise works as a stress reducer, helping you maintain mental well-being and limit the influence of stress on your diabetes.

F. Increased Energy Levels: Regular physical exercise enhances your overall energy levels. This may help alleviate symptoms of weariness that are occasionally connected with diabetes.

14.2 Exercise as a Mood Regulator

Exercise is not only excellent for physical health but also has a significant influence on mental health. The relationship between exercise and mood management is well-established:

A. Release of Endorphins: Exercise triggers the release of endorphins, which are natural mood lifters. This can help combat feelings of depression and anxiety, which are common among individuals with diabetes.

B. Stress Reduction: Engaging in physical activity reduces the production of stress hormones such as cortisol. Lower stress levels lead to improved mental well-being.

C. Improved Sleep: Regular exercise may aid with greater sleep quality. Quality sleep is vital for emotional stability and general mental wellness.

D. Enhanced Self-Esteem: As you get more physically fit and meet workout objectives, your self-esteem and self-confidence frequently receive a boost. This favorably influences your mental perspective.

E. Social engagement: Group workouts or team sports give chances for social engagement, lowering feelings of isolation and loneliness that patients with diabetes may experience.

14.3 Creating an Exercise Routine

Now that we understand the enormous advantages of exercise for diabetes and mental health, let's examine how to develop an exercise regimen that meets your needs:

A. Speak to a Healthcare practitioner: Before beginning any fitness regimen, speak with your healthcare practitioner. They can assist you in identifying the correct style and intensity of exercise for your unique condition.

B. Set Clear Goals: Determine what you want to accomplish with your training program. Whether it's better blood sugar management, weight reduction, or increased happiness, having clear objectives can keep you motivated.

C. Choose Activities You Enjoy: The finest fitness plan is one you'll stay with. Find activities you actually like, whether it's walking, swimming, dancing, or cycling.

D. Gradual Progression: Start softly and progressively raise the intensity and length of your exercises. This decreases the danger of damage and makes the habit more maintainable.

E. Consistency: Consistency is crucial. Aim for frequent, planned exercises. A combination of aerobic workouts (like walking or swimming) and strength training may be especially useful.

F. Monitor Your Blood Sugar: Keep a tight watch on your blood sugar levels before, during, and after exercise. This helps you understand how various activities influence your body.

G. Hydration and Nutrition: Stay hydrated and be cautious of your food. Proper eating is vital to fuel your exercise and maintain blood sugar levels.

H. Be Patient and Kind to Yourself: Progress may be sluggish, and there may be days when you don't feel like exercising. It's alright; don't be too harsh on yourself. Every effort counts.

In summary, exercise is a cornerstone of diabetes control and a strong tool for boosting mental well-being. When addressed with the correct mentality and supervision, an exercise regimen may greatly contribute to better blood sugar management, mood regulation, and improved overall quality of life for persons living with diabetes.

Chapter 15: Medications and Mental Health

Medications serve a vital part in diabetes care, helping patients regulate blood sugar levels. While they are vital for bodily health, it's critical to acknowledge their potential influence on mental well-being. This chapter discusses the relationship between diabetes drugs and mental health, highlighting the necessity of open communication with healthcare practitioners and ways for establishing a balance that assures both physical and mental wellness.

15.1 Medications for Diabetes and Their Effects on Mental Health

Living with diabetes frequently entails taking one or more medicines to manage blood sugar levels. These drugs are divided into numerous classes, including:

15.1.1 Insulin

Insulin is a hormone that helps control blood sugar. Many persons with type 1 diabetes and others with type 2 diabetes depend on insulin shots. The psychological elements of insulin usage include dread of injections, worry about dose estimates, and the danger of hypoglycemia (low blood sugar), which may lead to mood swings and anxiety.

15.1.2 Oral Medications

Oral medicines, such as metformin, sulfonylureas, and DPP-4 inhibitors, are routinely used to control type 2 diabetes. Some of these drugs may induce adverse effects including mood changes, gastrointestinal problems, or weight gain, which may influence mental health.

15.1.3 GLP-1 Receptor Agonists

GLP-1 receptor agonists are injectable drugs that assist in managing blood sugar and may contribute to weight reduction. They have been connected with increased mood and decreased symptoms of depression in certain people.

15.1.4 SGLT-2 Inhibitors

These drugs reduce blood sugar by helping the body eliminate extra glucose via urine. In certain situations, they may lead to urinary tract infections, which may damage mental well-being.

15.2 Communication with Healthcare Providers

Open and honest communication with healthcare professionals is vital when it comes to managing the interaction between diabetic drugs and mental health.

15.2.1 Establishing Trust

Building a trustworthy connection with your healthcare team is the first step. Share your problems, questions, and experiences connected to your medicine and mental health. They are there to assist you in discovering the best strategy for your scenario.

15.2.2 Medication Adjustments

If you discover that a certain medicine is impacting your mental health badly, discuss it with your healthcare practitioner. They might adapt their treatment plan or seek alternate drugs that may have fewer mental health adverse effects.

15.2.3 Mental Health Screening

Healthcare practitioners should frequently test persons with diabetes for mental health disorders since there is a significant correlation between the two. If you are having symptoms of sadness or anxiety, it's vital to mention them during your sessions.

15.2.4 Medication Education

Healthcare practitioners should give complete information about diabetic drugs, their possible adverse effects, and their influence on mental health. This helps people to make educated choices regarding their care.

15.3 Balancing Medication and Mental Well-being

Balancing the responsibilities of diabetes control and the possible effects of drugs on mental health may be tough, but it's vital for overall well-being.

15.3.1 Self-Monitoring

Regularly test your blood sugar levels to verify your medicine is appropriately controlling your diabetes. Feeling in control of your illness might significantly affect your mental health.

15.3.2 Lifestyle Modifications

Incorporate a healthy lifestyle that includes a balanced diet, frequent physical exercise, and stress management skills. These actions may help lessen the burden of diabetes and may enhance mental health.

15.3.3 Support Systems

Lean on your support network. Discuss your worries with friends and relatives. Join support groups to connect with people who understand the hardships of living with diabetes and the possible mental health implications of drugs.

15.3.4 Professional Help

Consider visiting a mental health expert if you encounter major mental health issues due to diabetes or its treatment. Therapy and counseling may give helpful coping methods and emotional support.

In conclusion, managing diabetes drugs and their influence on mental health is a multidimensional process that needs cooperation with healthcare practitioners, self-awareness, and a holistic approach to well-being. Recognizing the interaction between these two components and treating them proactively may lead to a better and more balanced existence for persons living with diabetes. Remember, you are not alone in this journey, and assistance is available to help you succeed both physically and psychologically.

Chapter 16: Supportive Therapies for Diabetes and Mental Health

Supportive treatments are an important component of addressing the complicated relationship between diabetes and mental health. In this chapter, we will cover three essential components of supportive treatments that may help persons with diabetes better their emotional well-being and general quality of life.

16.1 Psychotherapy and Counseling Options

Psychotherapy and counseling offer a secure and regulated setting for persons with diabetes to address their mental health difficulties. This sort of therapy includes talking to a skilled expert who can help you better understand your ideas, emotions, and actions. For patients with diabetes, psychotherapy may be especially effective in the following ways:

16.1.1 Understanding Emotional Triggers

Psychotherapy helps people to dive into the emotional causes that may impact their diabetes treatment. It helps you examine the psychological elements of living with a chronic disease, addressing difficulties such as fear, worry, and sadness. This knowledge is vital for building appropriate coping methods.

16.1.2 Cognitive-Behavioral Therapy (CBT)

CBT is a regularly utilized method of psychotherapy for patients with diabetes. It focuses on recognizing and modifying harmful thinking patterns and behaviors that might lead to mental health concerns. With CBT, you may learn to reframe negative ideas, manage stress, and increase self-control in diabetic self-care.

16.1.3 Diabetes-Specific Psychotherapy

Some therapists specialize in helping patients with diabetes manage the emotional elements of their illness. They may advise on concerns including fear of hypoglycemia, diabetes burnout, and diabetes-related anxiety. This tailored approach may make treatment more relevant and beneficial for persons with diabetes.

16.2 Group Therapy and Peer Support

Group therapy and peer support are effective tools for those with diabetes since they create a feeling of community and shared experiences. These techniques entail gathering with a group of folks who have similar difficulties, sometimes facilitated by a skilled facilitator. Here's how group therapy and peer support might assist persons with diabetes:

16.2.1 Shared Experiences

In a group environment, you'll encounter individuals who understand the particular difficulties of living with diabetes. Sharing experiences may minimize feelings of loneliness and help you obtain insights and coping skills from your peers.

16.2.2 Accountability

Group therapy and peer support may create a feeling of accountability. When you make objectives together, you may feel more driven to take better care of your diabetes and mental health.

16.2.3 Skill Building

Group therapy frequently focuses on improving certain abilities, such as stress management or problem-solving. These abilities are directly relevant to controlling diabetes and mental health concerns.

16.3 Integrative Approaches to Well-being

Integrative approaches to well-being target the full individual, including the physical, emotional, and spiritual components of health. These strategies may complement medical therapy and supporting interventions for persons with diabetes:

16.3.1 Mind-Body Practices

Mind-body therapies like yoga, tai chi, and meditation may enhance relaxation and stress reduction. They may also help manage blood sugar levels and promote general well-being.

16.3.2 Nutritional and Dietary Counseling

A proper diet is vital for diabetes treatment. Integrative health practitioners may give nutritional counseling targeted to your unique requirements, supporting improved blood sugar management and general health.

16.3.3 Complementary Therapies

Complementary treatments, such as acupuncture and massage, may help decrease diabetes-related discomfort and stress. While they should not replace medical therapy, they may be helpful complements to your care plan.

16.3.4 Holistic Lifestyle Changes

Integrative treatments frequently stress holistic lifestyle improvements. This includes increasing sleep, controlling stress, and adding physical exercise into your daily routine, all of which are critical for managing both diabetes and mental health.

In conclusion, the supportive treatments covered in this chapter offer vital tools for those living with diabetes and battling with mental health difficulties. These treatments provide diverse techniques to address the emotional elements of diabetes and promote general well-being. Whether via psychotherapy, group support, or integrative approaches, persons with diabetes have a choice of services to help them flourish emotionally and physically. Remember, it's crucial to engage with healthcare specialists to decide which tactics correspond best with your requirements and circumstances.

Chapter 17: Technology and Diabetes Management

As we journey farther into the 21st century, technology has revolutionized the way we manage chronic health issues like diabetes. This chapter discusses the changing landscape of technology improvements in diabetes treatment, the importance of applications and tools in providing mental health support, and the value of data management and monitoring in your diabetes journey.

17.1 Technological Advancements in Diabetes Care

Technology has changed diabetes treatment, bringing novel ways to enhance your everyday life and overall health. Here, we'll look into some of the most astonishing breakthroughs.

17.1.1 Continuous Glucose Monitoring (CGM) Systems

One of the most significant advancements in diabetes care is the emergence of Continuous Glucose Monitoring (CGM) devices. These gadgets continually measure your blood glucose levels, delivering real-time data without the need for frequent finger pricking. They give insights into your glucose patterns, letting you make educated decisions regarding your dietary choices, medicine, and physical activity.

17.1.2 Insulin Pumps

Insulin pumps have changed throughout the years, becoming more user-friendly and effective. These devices give a continuous supply of insulin, closely imitating the function of a functioning pancreas. With features like automated modifications based on CGM data, they enable improved glycemic control, minimizing the risk of severe highs and lows.

17.1.3 Artificial Pancreas Systems

Artificial pancreas devices offer a huge breakthrough in diabetes technology. These closed-loop devices integrate CGM data with insulin pump technology to automatically adjust insulin supply, delivering improved stability and lowering the stress of ongoing monitoring and decision-making.

17.1.4 Telemedicine and Virtual Care

Telemedicine and virtual care have become crucial tools in diabetes treatment, giving the ease of remote consultations with healthcare specialists. These platforms offer frequent check-ins, revisions to your treatment plan, and access to professional assistance from the comfort of your own home.

17.2 Apps and Tools for Mental Health Support

Mental health is a vital element of diabetes care, and various applications and programs are intended to give you the support you need.

17.2.1 Meditation and Relaxation Apps

Managing diabetes may be stressful, and stress can alter blood sugar levels. Meditation and relaxation applications lead you through mindfulness activities, helping you decrease stress and anxiety. Regular practice might enhance your overall mental well-being.

17.2.2 Diabetes Diary Apps

Keeping note of your everyday events and feelings associated with diabetes might be vital for your mental health. Diabetes diary applications enable you to document your meals, exercise, blood sugar levels, and mood. This data may help you uncover trends and triggers, leading to enhanced emotional well-being.

17.2.3 Support Groups and Forums

Online support groups and forums give a place to interact with others experiencing similar issues. Sharing experiences, worries, and triumphs may be a vital source of emotional support. These groups build a sense of belonging and alleviate feelings of loneliness.

17.2.4 Mindfulness and Cognitive Behavioral Therapy (CBT) Apps

Mindfulness and CBT applications are meant to help you manage stress, anxiety, and depression. They give participatory activities and ways to improve resilience and deal with the emotional elements of diabetes.

17.3 Data Management and Tracking

Data is a significant tool in diabetes care, helping you to make educated choices and discover patterns. Proper data management is vital for a successful diabetes journey.

17.3.1 Blood Glucose Tracking

Regular monitoring of blood glucose levels is crucial. There are many technologies, like as digital glucose meters and CGM systems, that deliver reliable readings. Tracking your glucose levels helps you learn how your body reacts to diverse circumstances including diet, exercise, and medication.

17.3.2 Food and Nutrition Apps

Diet plays a significant part in controlling diabetes. Food and nutrition applications allow you to track your meals, count carbs, and manage your calorie consumption. They may also give nutritional information, helping you make better eating choices.

17.3.3 Medication and Insulin Dosing Apps

For patients on various medicines or insulin regimens, pharmaceutical and insulin dosage applications may simplify the procedure. They remind you to take your meds and calculate insulin dosages, lowering the risks of mistakes.

17.3.4 Health Records and Cloud Storage

Managing your health data might be intimidating, but technology provides alternatives. Health record applications and cloud storage alternatives enable you to organize and securely keep your medical information, making them conveniently available for healthcare practitioners and emergencies.

In conclusion, technology has become an invaluable ally in the complicated terrain of diabetes treatment. From sophisticated monitoring systems to mental health support applications and data management tools, the incorporation of technology helps those with diabetes to lead better lives. Embracing these developments may make the trip more bearable and give crucial support for both your physical and emotional well-being.

Chapter 18: Diabetes and Aging

As people age, the treatment of diabetes takes on a new set of complications. This chapter discusses the many facets of aging with diabetes and gives helpful advice on how to properly navigate this era of life. Managing diabetes in older persons involves a comprehensive strategy that takes into consideration physical health, cognitive changes, and the maintenance of overall quality of life.

18.1 Managing Diabetes in Older Adults

Managing diabetes in older persons is a difficult endeavor that takes a combination of medical expertise, lifestyle modifications, and a thorough awareness of the individual's particular requirements. This section will look into the important factors and solutions for properly controlling diabetes in the elderly.

18.1.1 Individualized Care Plans

The first step in controlling diabetes in older persons is to construct personalized treatment plans. Each person's requirements and abilities may differ, so it's vital to work closely with healthcare experts to build a tailored diabetes treatment strategy. This plan should incorporate issues such as current health concerns, medication management, food choices, and physical activity levels.

18.1.2 Medication Management

Elderly persons with diabetes typically need many drugs to regulate their blood sugar. Managing these drugs may be tough, so it's crucial to ensure a healthcare professional frequently checks and modifies the prescription regimen as required. Avoiding drug interactions and adverse effects is crucial at this time of life.

18.1.3 Nutrition and Diet

Nutrition has a key role in treating diabetes, and this is particularly true for older persons. Monitoring carbohydrate consumption, portion sizes, and meal time is critical. Nutritionists or dietitians may assist in constructing a balanced meal plan that takes into consideration individual dietary preferences and any required alterations.

18.1.4 Physical Activity and Mobility

Maintaining physical exercise, even in a restricted form, is critical for treating diabetes in older persons. Exercise helps enhance insulin sensitivity, muscular strength, and general health. Healthcare practitioners may propose safe and acceptable physical activities depending on an individual's talents and limits.

18.1.5 Regular Monitoring

Regular monitoring of blood glucose levels is crucial to measure the efficiency of the treatment strategy. This may require daily glucose checks, HbA1c testing, and frequent check-ups with healthcare specialists. Adjustments may be made based on these monitoring data.

18.1.6 Coordination of Care

Elderly adults generally have a network of healthcare professionals, including primary care doctors, endocrinologists, and specialists for various health concerns. Coordinating care among various specialists is vital to guarantee that the overall health of the person is handled successfully.

18.2 Cognitive Changes in Aging with Diabetes

As people age, they may have cognitive changes, and this might provide special issues while controlling diabetes. In this part, we study the relationship between diabetes and cognitive performance in older persons.

18.2.1 Cognitive Aging

Cognitive aging is a normal process where certain cognitive skills may diminish with age. These alterations may include slower processing speed, diminished working memory, and decreased attention span. Diabetes may worsen these changes, making it vital to alter diabetes care measures appropriately.

18.2.2 Hypoglycemia Awareness

Hypoglycemia (low blood sugar) may have a major influence on cognitive performance. Older persons may suffer lower awareness of hypoglycemia symptoms, making it necessary to check blood sugar levels regularly. Family members and caregivers should also be taught about spotting indicators of hypoglycemia.

18.2.3 Medication Management and Cognitive Function

Some diabetic drugs may impact cognitive performance, especially in elderly persons. Healthcare practitioners should consider the cognitive side effects of drugs when picking the most suitable treatment choices for aged patients.

18.2.4 Cognitive Impairment and Self-Care

Cognitive disability, such as dementia, might affect diabetes control. Family members and caregivers may need to take a more active role in aiding persons with cognitive impairments in their regular self-care activities.

18.3 Maintaining Quality of Life in Later Years

Maintaining quality of life is a vital priority for older persons with diabetes. This section covers several techniques to increase the general well-being of older adults while controlling their diabetes.

18.3.1 Emotional Support

Emotional well-being is vital to quality of life. Older adults may face emotional challenges related to the physical limitations and lifestyle changes necessitated by diabetes. Support from family members, friends, and mental health professionals can help individuals cope with these challenges.

18.3.2 Social Engagement

Staying socially engaged is vital for mental and emotional health. Encouraging older persons to engage in social activities, support groups, and community events may contribute to a higher quality of life.

18.3.3 End-of-Life Planning

End-of-life planning is a difficult but crucial concern for older persons with diabetes. Discussing preferences for care, advanced directives, and end-of-life choices with family and healthcare professionals may bring peace of mind and guarantee the individual's desires are honored.

18.3.4 Adaptation and Resilience

Adaptation and resilience are key skills while controlling diabetes in older years. Learning to adapt to changes, bounce back from failures, and discover new sources of pleasure and purpose may considerably increase an individual's quality of life.

In conclusion, this chapter underlines the particular issues experienced by older persons with diabetes and presents a detailed roadmap to handle these challenges. By emphasizing tailored treatment, addressing cognitive changes, and promoting overall well-being, older persons may continue to lead happy lives while successfully managing their diabetes.

Chapter 19: Family and Caregiver Support

Living with diabetes, especially when it is connected to mental health difficulties, can be a journey filled with ups and downs. In this chapter, we discuss the critical role that family members and caregivers play in assisting persons struggling with diabetes and its influence on mental health. We will go into understanding the significance of the family's role, effective strategies to offer assistance and the equally crucial notion of self-care for caregivers.

19.1 The Role of Family in Diabetes and Mental Health

Diabetes and mental health problems may be daunting for people afflicted, and family members are generally the first source of assistance. Let's take a deeper look at the essential function that family plays in this scenario.

19.1.1 Understanding the Emotional Impact

Dealing with a chronic disease like diabetes may provoke a broad variety of feelings, including anxiety, frustration, and grief. When mental health is also at risk, these feelings might worsen. Family members should notice and comprehend these emotional effects on their loved ones.

19.1.2 Providing Emotional Support

A caring and understanding family may help minimize the emotional strain on someone with diabetes and mental health difficulties. Listen actively, give a shoulder to rely on, and establish an atmosphere where frank talks about emotions are encouraged.

19.1.3 Involvement in Treatment

Families may actively engage in the diabetes and mental health treatment process. This involves attending medical visits, understanding prescription regimes, and partnering with healthcare experts to offer the best treatment possible.

19.1.4 Education and Advocacy

Becoming well-informed on diabetes and its link to mental health is vital. Families may advocate for their loved ones by educating themselves, creating awareness, and campaigning for greater healthcare access and support systems.

19.2 Providing Effective Support

Being helpful is not always uncomplicated. To give appropriate assistance to someone with diabetes and mental health difficulties, consider the following:

19.2.1 Encourage Healthy Lifestyle Choices

Support people in making healthy decisions about nutrition, exercise, and medication adherence. Encouragement and involvement in these activities may be immensely inspiring.

19.2.2 Assist in Blood Sugar Monitoring

Help with monitoring blood glucose levels, particularly when mental health difficulties make self-care tough. This assistance may avoid hazardous swings in blood sugar.

19.2.3 Promote Stress Management

Stress is a crucial component impacting both diabetes and mental health. Encourage stress-reduction practices such as mindfulness, relaxation exercises, or hobbies that offer pleasure.

19.2.4 Offer Non-Judgmental Understanding

Living with diabetes and mental health difficulties is already tough. Avoid blame, criticism, or judgment. Instead, provide understanding, tolerance, and love.

19.3 Self-Care for Caregivers

Caregivers frequently forget to take care of themselves while focused on their loved ones. However, self-care is crucial to ensure that carers can continue to offer assistance efficiently.

19.3.1 Recognizing Caregiver Stress

It's typical for carers to endure stress and exhaustion. Recognize the indicators of caregiver stress, which may include weariness, worry, and disregard for one's health.

19.3.2 Seeking Support and Resources

Caregivers should not hesitate to seek help from support groups, therapists, or other caregivers who can relate to their experiences. Resources are available to assist carers in maintaining their well-being.

19.3.3 Time Management and Boundaries

Establish limits and manage time wisely to minimize caregiver burnout. This can require obtaining respite care or support from other family members to split the tasks.

19.3.4 Self-Care Activities*

Engage in self-care activities that enhance mental and emotional well-being, such as exercise, meditation, hobbies, or just taking time for relaxation.

In this chapter, we've studied the essential role of family in assisting those with diabetes and mental health difficulties. Effective support encompasses understanding, encouragement, active engagement in therapy, and education. Additionally, carers must remember to take care of themselves, recognize their stress, and seek help when required. This holistic approach helps provide a friendly and loving atmosphere that may enhance the overall well-being of persons living with diabetes and mental health difficulties.

Chapter 20: Looking Forward: Thriving with Diabetes and Mental Health

Living with diabetes while maintaining excellent mental health is a journey that involves perseverance, drive, and a positive mindset. In this last chapter, we will study the art of flourishing with diabetes and mental health. We'll address how developing a positive mentality, creating long-term objectives, and the future of diabetes treatment and mental health integration may contribute to a meaningful and balanced life despite the hurdles.

20.1 Embracing a Positive Outlook

Living with diabetes may be hard, but it's crucial to retain a positive mindset to better manage the illness. Here, we'll dig into the significance of a positive mentality and present practical ideas on how to embrace it.

20.1.1 The Power of Positivity

An optimistic mindset may dramatically improve your general well-being. It may lower stress, improve blood sugar regulation, and promote your mental wellness. Positivity is not about dismissing the hardships of diabetes but accepting them and finding positive methods to cope with them.

20.1.2 Cultivating Positivity

Practice gratitude: Regularly reflect on the things you're glad for, no matter how minor. This might change your emphasis from the issues to the good in your life.

Surround yourself with support: Engage with friends, family, or support groups that understand your path. Sharing experiences may build a feeling of belonging and happiness.

Mindfulness and meditation: These activities may help you remain present and manage stress, creating a more hopeful view.

20.2 Setting Long-Term Goals

Setting meaningful long-term objectives is a critical element of living with diabetes and mental health. It provides you with purpose, direction, and drive to take charge of your health.

20.2.1 Why Set Long-Term Goals?

Long-term objectives create a feeling of purpose, helping you to look beyond everyday problems. They might include increasing blood sugar management, decreasing weight, or learning a new skill.

These objectives help you remain motivated and resilient.

20.2.2 How to Set Effective Goals

Specific: Clearly explain your aims. For example, "I want to reduce my A1c levels by 1% over the next year."

Measurable: Ensure you can monitor your development. Use tools like a blood glucose monitor or diary to maintain records.

Achievable: Make sure your objectives are reasonable. They should push you yet stay reachable.

Relevant: Goals should correspond with your entire well-being and values. They should matter to you.

Time-bound: Set a deadline to generate a feeling of urgency and keep you focused.

20.3 The Future of Diabetes Care and Mental Health Integration

As medical research progresses, the future of diabetes treatment and mental health integration appears hopeful. The healthcare environment is shifting to better serve patients living with both diabetes and mental health challenges.

20.3.1 Holistic Care Approach

Healthcare professionals are increasingly embracing a holistic approach to treatment. This involves acknowledging that physical and mental health are intertwined. You should anticipate more individualized treatment strategies that target both your diabetes and mental health concerns.

20.3.2 Technological Advancements

Technology is playing a vital role in diabetes control and mental health assistance.

Innovations like continuous glucose monitoring (CGM) and telemedicine services enable improved tracking, communication, and management.

20.3.3 Psychosocial Support

Mental health treatments and support networks are becoming increasingly accessible. You may expect more availability of mental health experts who are educated to assist with those managing diabetes.

20.3.4 Research and Advocacy

The future also offers potential in terms of research and campaigning. Diabetes and mental health groups are trying to promote awareness and lobby for legislation that enhances the lives of persons afflicted by both disorders.

In conclusion, living with diabetes and keeping excellent mental health is not only conceivable but a realistic objective. By adopting a positive mindset, creating important long-term objectives, and looking forward to the future of integrated care, you may lead a satisfying life despite the obstacles provided by diabetes and its influence on mental health. Remember, you're not alone, and the route to flourishing with diabetes and mental health is one filled with hope, strength, and support.

www.ingramcontent.com/pod-product-compliance
Lightning Source LLC
Chambersburg PA
CBHW050819260726

48660CB00004B/1518